2018

SOUS VIDE at KITCHEN

THE VACUUM TECHNIQUE FOR QUALITY COOKED MEALS

JOAN ANDERSON

Table of Contents

Introduction

If you like to carry out amazing experiments in the kitchen, you have probably heard or even used to cook dishes sous vide. Many famous restaurants all over the world use the method of sous vide to reach the special tenderness, flavor and delicious taste of the ingredients that we eat every day. It is an alternative way of cooking ingredients that allows reaching an incredibly juicy meat, poultry or chicken, saving all necessary microelements and vitamins. The boring days of chewy steak or chicken have already gone. Today is time to enjoy moist and tender food with colorful vegetables. Frying or roasting food we may get it overcooked or still raw food inside. Sous vide method allows cooking ingredients through even by low temperature and only after this process you may brown or sear the ingredients if needed. Of course, it may sound too good to be real, but sous vide method has been already experienced not only by chefs of the famous restaurants all over the world but also by thousands of housekeepers.

Using sous vide in your kitchen is a great tool that units the following advantages – exact temperature control of readiness; tender texture of food in comparison with traditional cooking methods; lowering of pathogens to a no-effect level using the low temperature; the process of vacuum evaporation prolongs the preservation of the ingredients and reduces the possible risk of recontamination, keeps the natural flavors and escapes the loss of essential elements.

Today many people are busy. Our usual working days begins with a thought that we have to do a crazy list of actions today and, probably, too many troubles to think what and how to cook the steak of meat. Cooking dishes sous vide makes us free from the worries what, how and when to cook the dishes for our family and how to eat healthy food. This book reveals you a secret what is sous vide actually, what tools do you need to cook sous vide and, moreover, the book presents you a step-by-step guide of the recipes of your favorite dishes cooked sous vide.

What is sous vide cooking?

Sous vide... This sounds powerful than it is in reality. The popular combination fascinates the thoughts of thousands of experts and cooking fans, taking parts in the cooking shows and world competitions of the chefs. What is this method of cooking about? Do the chefs of the popular restaurants in the world use this technique? What is the sous vide technique really about? Sous vide that is translated as "under vacuum" in French, is a popular cooking technique that applies exact temperature control to perform high quality, respective results. It means, in general, the usual process of the vacuum-sealing products in a bag, then cooking it to a very exact temperature in a heated water bath, with no connection of a heated steel surface. There is also no connection with flames or smoke. Moreover, the water can't come to a boil. Yeah, it's a great discovery! This method of cooking foods shows unbelievable results that are insufferable to attain using any other cooking technique. The popular restaurants of the world use the method of the sous vide to prepare food for the stated level of preparedness. This mode of preparation has got a success at home preparation with the facility of conceivable and easy-to-use sous vide specific cooking equipment.

The equipment of sous vide applies the heated metal helical to heat up the water to a necessary temperature, keeping the balance between too high or extremely low temperatures. It means that the preparation advance is successive and adjustable. Such full-proteins pieces like pork, fish or chicken are always prepared for long periods of time, heated up very slowly, step by step until the complete piece attains the same temperature as the water. We have already mentioned, the water never goes past the wishful temperature of readiness, so the piece of meat takes notably longer preparation time. But! Everything has its pros and cons and preparing food this way you'll never have the over boiled food. Remember the situation, when the same piece of meat is cooked by you on the stove, the direct heat you use brings the inside temperature of approximately 135°F. At this time it is almost impossible (or you may just guess) what is going on inside the piece of meat. When you cut the piece of meat you'll get the damaged presentation of your dish, otherwise, you'll not see if it is ready or not. Using the method of sous vide, there are no inconveniences at all. Everything is so simple – when you put the piece of meat in a heated bath, there is no chance that the food will be overcooked or go past the wished temperature. The water circulation, the next magical function of the sous vide, allows reaching the medium-rare throughout. Your piece of meat that is prepared in sous vide technique will not be caramelized, crispy or even charred because of the absence of the contact with the surface. Roasting meat like pork or steak in a heated skillet for a minute from each side allows getting the *caramelization* without cooking the whole piece of meat from inside. Moreover, you need all the time being present in the kitchen and checking the cooking temperature, turn the pieces of meat from start to finish. Sous vide technique saves your time, allows to serve and slice quickly by providing the 100 percent of the inside readiness of foods.

You may say that you are not a restaurant chef and you have no reason to cook sous vide. But what if I remember you about saving time and lazy weekend dinners? Do you want to rat around in the kitchen while the other family members are outside or to be together with the crowd? Less time spending on a stove; you may keep the cooked foods in the fridge for a whole week. No stress at all. Sous vide takes care of your family budget – the cheaper cuts could get tender and tastier.

What do people love sous vide?

The technique of sous vide has become popular because of great delicious tastes and an amazing hands-off way of preparing. The natural juices of foods and flavors are the results of the slow and gentle cooking technique that doesn't need much attention. It is the healthiest way to cook foods in comparison to preparation methods that need added fat, medium or high heat that breaks down in any way the healthy components of products. This method of cooking could be widely used for such dishes like vegetables, grains, meat, custard, beans etc. where different foods need their special temperatures to be fully cooked through. Using this way of cooking make you free from being dependent typical recipes that utilize the usual stove, oven, and grill. The needed preparation time for finality is set by a wide array of variables, like the cookware, stove, and the way, for example, you always control the heat.

The procedure of preparation applying this method is simply easy, the following steps let you get the overall concept of the process:

1. Arranging the temperature - this manner permits controlling over the strict temperature you will need for preparing the products. For example, when you confer a toasted medium-rare slab of meat to a braised stew. In general, the steak is crude, mostly of red color and could be even a little bit rubber like. The pot roast is of brown color, a little dry and is soft pull-apart. All the slabs of meat with various readiness, even those that are all "medium-rare" are still the same type of dish, in general, especially when they are conferred to the pot roast. The medium-rare type is from approximately 130°F to 139°F (or 54°C to 59°C). Some absolute sous vide points are: medium beef: 140°F-145°F, extra-juicy tender pork: 135°F-145°F, classic tender pork: 145°F-155°F, classic chicken breast: 140°F-150°F, classic fish: 122°F-132°F. So choosing a point is rather simple, it depends on what kind of meat or fish you want.
2. Heat up the water – I think you know many different methods to heat up the water for sous vide preparation. Fortunately, there are some cost-friendly methods that are available and that you can simply use with sous vide technique without spending a lot of money.
3. Seal the food in a bag - This stage saves the peculiarity of the food you will be cook applying the sous vide way. The most forceful way of sealing products is utilizing a located vacuum sealer. But pay attention, they are too valuable as well as commonly excessively for domestic use. Instead of this, you may use the famous Ziploc Freezer Bags that work great for most products.
4. Arranging the duration – There is the main aim when you will arrange the prolongation of preparing the products, whether using sous vide or following classical way. The computation of time of fully heating the products is rather easy following sous vide technique on the occasion of the heated water bath is at an initial temperature. It usually takes you approximately about an hour for a 1" thick piece of meat and, for example, 3 hours for a 2" thick piece to heat fully. As contrasted with classical preparation processes, the sous vide method admits

food to escape being overcooked within the process. Using the wide-spread way of sous vide you must follow the next rule: tenderize the products – people usually cook foods that are rather delicate such as fish, chicken, steaks that just need to be heated fully. But still, there are a lot of kinds of meat that require tenderization. The longer you prepare your favorite products following sous vide method the more delicate food you get. The general and the easiest difference of this is that adding time to sous vide preparing doesn't digest your food. The sous vide point is rather low, that's why the tenderization procedure comes more inertly, arising with long length cooking times.

5. Finish cooking process with a sear – the main thing of a tasty, amazing dish is the crunchy, fragrant layer that you can become after usual preparation procedure using the skillet or the saucepan. But sadly, this is the thing that the sous vide doesn't do, no crunch layers at all. But! You may sear the already prepared foods on a hot grill, using a burner, or even fry it, any method that is most appropriated for you and your guests.

Why Should I Sous Vide?

The sous vide method is the wide-spread common way of preparing tasty and healthy dishes at home. By putting the ingredients in a plastic bag, discharging the air and preparing the ingredients in a heated water bath and saving the free time, one may get incredible meals. I think it is already the reason to try the sous vide method, but, of course, it is not the only simple reason you should run to the kitchen and begin with cooking (but, still you may). There a lot of them:

1. I think, there are a lot of women (and men also) who have tried the difficult way of cooking their best meals and keep in a secret their family recipes. Still, everybody has heard the old stories from the mothers, how the grandmothers have cooked these dishes at their best and tried to do it until they were dead. Sometimes, it is too hard to follow somebodies recipe and prepare it as well as the mother or granny cooked it. In most cases, the first endeavor is always unlucky – the meal is mostly overcooked or damp. But how do I get the juicy meat of fish? Using the sous vide method you have the option of the temperature control at which the ingredients are cooked, but they never get dry – even if a person prefers them well done! They could be perfectly well-cooked but still juicy and flavorful. Even if someone leaves the ingredients in the water bath longer than the mentioned amount of time, sometimes even for hours, the ingredients will not be overcooked or chewy. The guidelines may help the beginner to maintain the textural integrity of the food a person cooks.

2. Sous vide saves the budget – you will ask me *Why*? And the answer is rather simple – because your flank steak will taste like a filet mignon! You will cook the restaurant dishes at home that could save your money. Those who use sous vide are able to buy the cheaper meat parts or chicken and prepare them more delicious than ever! And no other investments from your pocket! Preparing the ingredients in a closed vacuum bag, the humid environment created there will braise the meat essentially. Finally, you'll get amazing five-star dishes!

3. Sous vide cooking is safer – everyone who prefers to cook or even those who do not have burned themselves several times. The process of cooking involves usage of different equipment, fire, and cook under hot temperatures. Being all the time in a hurry, we may burn ourselves very often paying no attention to flames, heated skillets that are painful and dangerous. Using the sous vide method one chooses the necessary temperature that is between 40ºC and 85ºC and that's all, so, you don't need to use flame, heated skillets or other dangerous kitchen equipment.

4. Kids like getting involved with the method of sous vide – this point is of high importance for women and especially for housekeepers as they always have no time either for kids no for cooking. But! This time the parents must be really surprised as the kids like to be involved in the procedure of sous vide and, of course, eating their creations! As we have already mentioned, this process is safety, that's why they are ready to help you in the kitchen all the time. Putting the ingredients into the bath could be a perfect job to help mother or granny. The several researchers have shown that kids that are involved in cooking meals at home or helping someone cooking, make out of the home the healthier choices than their

counterparts that are not involved in cooking processes at home. The kids enjoy also the texture of vegetables and meats, wonder of cooking equipment.

5. Cooking sous vide requires less fat, oil, and salt than traditional cooking ways we use every day. The slow-cooking process keeps more nutrients and makes them in this way more accessible. It can help a person to accommodate special diets and forget about a range of problems. Cooking food in a vacuum seal means that all the natural juices and vitamins are saved, they are not boiled off or steamed away like in conventional cooking, the meals that are prepared by sous vide way keep their color and form. One should not need to add butter or oils to moisten dry meat or vegetables. The natural flavors are enhanced by this method of foods preparation.

6. Everybody can sous vide almost anywhere – using sous vide method you don't need to use all the kitchen area and a lot of places. Everything you need is an electrical outlet, a supply of water and a container. Don't forget about the ingredients, of course! Some persons travel a lot and take all necessary appliances to be sure they are eating healthy, delicious meals wherever they go.

7. Sous vide cooking method is low maintenance – Preparing meals sous vide does not require excessive amounts of attention. A person who is cooking does not need to be standing all the time over a hot stove just to be sure that the ingredients do not burn; one just heats the bath, drops the food in, and sets the timer. You may also use the handy app, hearing the alarm a person knows that food is ready. But if you don't want, you may not to use an app – you can keep it as simple as you please. All the people have bad days in the kitchen- the ingredients get burned and tempers get frayed. Using the sous vide method one follows a very precise temperature, that's why it is really very hard to mess up. If somebody isn't very good at cooking – it is not a problem! Sous vide method is as easy to use as a microwave.

8. Less dirty dishes – cooking the sous vide method means that you use fewer dirty dishes. Yes! It is an amazing point for women and everybody who doesn't like to wash it! Sometimes, especially if a person has a too busy day, there is no time to wash the dishes at all! Using the sous vide technique you may cook the meat or fish and get too little washing up to do after the whole process. You may eat the dish at once after the cooking time is over or sear it for some minutes in a pan.

9. Sous vide is a great method to make-ahead meals – using this technique people may easily prepare for a whole week or even for a month! Could you imagine this? Some women are always afraid of buying, for example, a package of chicken on sale. Now, you don't worry about this! It is very easy, because you divide and portion the meat out however you choose to cook them in the marinade, freeze or something else. Using the sous vide method you may easily prepare the dishes for the whole busy week and keep them in the fridge!

10. Incredible device – I hope, that you have already understood, that using the sous vide technique you will save the electricity in comparison to many other kitchen appliances that will also save your money. Moreover, you will not feel yourself like a furnace while cooking some dishes simultaneously in the kitchen on a hot day.

11. One can appeal to a number of palates at the same time – this was always a problem! For example, a mother prefers her steak with simply salt and pepper, and no more species! A father wants his steak with hot chili. A daughter likes the same piece of meat but with Italian Seasoning and the Worcestershire sauce. And all they want to eat together at the same time. Is this possible? Yes! Of course! Different dishes in the same water bath! Could you imagine!? It is also possible to manage various degrees of readiness perfectly with a little extra time spent cooking. This will make both family dinner and a dinner party less stressful. And if you will choose the recipes carefully, you will be able to cook different recipes at the same time.

12. Meal planning for healthy eating - If someone is preparing something like lamb chops or steaks, why not cooking some extra pieces for use another time. Everything is so simple! After you'll have some extra steaks, you may easily freeze them and then grill quickly when you will need.

13. Makes gourmet cooking look easy – the sous vide technique that is widely used in the restaurants makes gourmet cooking easy. Some of your preferred recipes seem to be impossible to cook at home. You have tried too many times, toasted, stewed or baked them but as a result – you get the damaged ingredients and lose money and time. This time, using the sous vide technique you will be surprised as none of the recipes could be damaged at all.

14. Impressing guests – Sometimes we try to surprise our guests with new dishes, searching on the Internet for hours trying to find something easy in cooking but tasty. We buy expensive ingredients and skillets, saucepans and grillers to reach the wished consistency. But it happens that the guests are already in the kitchen but the dinner is fully ruined! Following the sous vide method you'll get the ready dinner or supper before the guests are already by you! When the guests of family members only taste the sous vide cooked food, they will be going to be surprised!

So, I think, this is enough pros to ensure you to try this new and exciting method of cooking.

Tools & Techniques

After you have understood what the technique of sous vide really is, let's try to understand what the tools you need.

1. Vacuum sealing sacks

First of all – what is vacuum sealing in general? This method can actually renew the tenability up to three times. It is of high importance that one can use the vacuum sealer sacks correctly. When utilizing sous vide, the bags are the primary tool a person needs to buy. It is necessary to realize, that not every sealing bag corresponds to each vacuum sealer. So, that's why a person has to buy the exact one he/she needs.

The sealers are of two kinds mostly – the chamber and bar sealers. The sealers could be found in almost all shops for kitchen equipment and tools. The bar sealers work traditionally by a simple absorbing - intake approach when a person places food into the special bag after this set the bag under the bar and finally, the sealing machine absorbs the air. The bar sealers are not allowed to be utilized with redundant fluid, as this kind of sealer would intake the fluid further into the air.

To utilize the fluids with the sealer:

1. you may freeze the fluid in an ice cube and put to a sack.

2. you may utilize a renowned ziplock bag.

The chamber sealers (the second type) could be utilized with fluids. It is enabled to cook innovative and distinctive dishes. While the bar sealers intake air right from the sack, the chamber sealers eliminate the air from all the field. They produce a void space that seals and condense the sack at the same time.

The vacuum process includes the following steps:

1. Fill the sack (vacuum bag) with components.
2. Tighten the bar sealer onto the open end of the vacuum sack and switch on the appliance.
3. Remove the sack which has already been packed.

Speaking about finishing steps of preparing the recipes sous vide, one should know the following rule: Once the preparation time is over, one should carefully take off the cooked food from the sack (it is hot!), let it cool a little and in order to remove the rest unnecessary fluid dry with a paper towel the sack. After the first step of preparing sous vide (when it is fish, meat or etc.) you may roast them a little bit to get the wished crispy.

2. Thermometer

When you have finally decided to prepare some dishes sous vide, it is of high importance to be aware of what food and water temperature you must have. This is the reason a person needs a thermometer. The special thermometer is traditionally designed for preparing sous vide, so you may easily see the temperature of the ingredients of a vacuum sack. The band permits a user to pick the sack with the spicule probe of the thermometer. Don't be afraid of losing money if you make investments in the thermometer but don't cook sous vide rather often. It is a necessary part of kitchen tools you may need all the time. There are multiple prices of the thermometers that will allow you to see the temperature of food in a sack.

3. Vacuum condenser

The vacuum condensers are exploited as a conceivable device to vacuum the components. The condensers usually intake the air out of the vacuum sack. Just put the open edge of your vacuum sack downside the cover of the sealer which will draw out the air and seals with heat.

4. Water container

After you have bought almost all the necessary devices to utilize sous vide at home, everything you need at the end is water case that you need to warm up the water to the necessary temperature.

The easiest method of how to warm up the water is to utilize the water case. When utilizing the water oven, both of the elements - the case and the heating set cooperate as one. The water oven is one of the best conclusions for those who want to prepare recipes sous vide at home and also who doesn't want to buy a lot of equipment. The water container allows checking the temperature easily. The other method that is also possible is to use a thermal circulator with case together. Such circulators allow warming up the water with high exactness: to check the temperature standing upon the volume of the pot you joined. It is highly recommended to choose a case with a lid because it guaranties gained insolation and ensures that water will not come through evaporation.

Vegetarian & Vegan

Sous vide Deonjang-Spiced aubergine

When you are bored with old recipes and usual vegetables that are you can buy every day in the nearest store, give them a little bit Korean taste and amazing flavor. Don't forget to use the sous vide technique!

Ingredients (6 servings):

4 Pieces	Thai aubergine
1/4 Cup	vegetable oil
2 Tbsp	Deonjang paste
2 Tbsp	Soy sauce
1 Tbsp	Brown sugar
1 Tbsp	Sesame seeds

Pepper and salt at will

Directions:
1. Wash and dry with a paper towel the aubergines. Cut them into pieces.
2. Take a small bowl, whisk the Deonjang paste together with peanut oil, add soy sauce, and also the brown sugar.
3. Add the aubergines into the same bowl. Mix everything thoroughly.
4. Put the sauce and the aubergines into a sous vide bag.
5. Cook for 35-45 minutes at 185F.
6. After the time is over, drain the rest of the aubergine wedges from the liquid.
7. Take a medium-sized skillet, heat it a little and sear the aubergines in it.
8. Top with the rest of sesame seeds before eating.
9. Bon Appetite!

Sous vide garlic chili Tofu

An amazing and delicious recipe using Tofu slices that are really full of Asian flavor. I advise you to serve them with Asian rice or other green veggies.

Ingredients (5 servings):

1 Block	Firm Tofu
1/4 Cup	Soy Sauce
1/2 Cup	Brown Sugar
1/4 Cup	Sesame Oil
2 Tablespoons	Chili-Garlic Paste

Pepper and salt to taste

Basil leaves for garnish

Directions:
1. Open the bag with a firm piece of Tofu and slice into big blocks.
2. Take a medium-sized skillet and roast a little bit the Tofu slices for some minutes until they become a golden color.
3. Take a large bowl, put the Tofu slice on a bottom, add soy sauce, sugar, sprinkle with sesame oil, add the paste.
4. Toss everything to coat the Tofu slices. Be careful not to damage the slices.
5. Put the slices into the sous vide bag, add sauce and cook for approximately 4 hours at 180F.
6. Serve in a large plate. Garnish with some fresh basil leaves.
7. Bon Appetite!

French fries sous vide

This is an amazing recipe for cooking French fries through the sous vide method. I think, everybody like this. Try to cook French fries in a new way.

Ingredients (5 servings):

500 Grams   Potatoes

1/2 Cup   Water

1/2 Tbsp   Salt

1/4 Tbsp   Sugar

1/4 Tsp   Baking Soda

avocado oil for frying

Salt and pepper at will

Directions:
1. Wash and peel carefully potatoes. After this, cut into half-inch batons or another way you prefer.
2. In a medium-sized bowl conjoin together salt, water, baking soda, and sugar.
3. Put the batons into a sous vide bag adding the mixture.
4. Close and cook for circa 15 minutes at 190F.
5. Air dry the vegetables.
6. Take a medium-sized skillet, add the oil and fry quickly the potatoes for 6 minutes at 125F.
7. Drain from the rest of oil and let them cook.
8. Season quickly with pepper and salt at will.
9. Eat warm!

Sous vide sunchokes with toasted almonds

Have you ever tried to cook the sunchokes? Have you tried to cook them using sous vide? This time I combine both the sunchokes and the sous vide technique. You will be surprised with the result!

Ingredients (3 servings):

1 1/2 pounds   sunchokes

4 Tbsp   olive oil

2 Tbsp   almonds

fresh chives

salt and black pepper if desired

Directions:
1. Set the sous vide cooker to 190°F.
2. Scrabble the sunchokes, put them in a sealed bag, don't forget to sprinkle with pepper. Add salt.
3. Add the oil. Seal the bag.
4. Put the bag in the water bath and set the timer for 1 hour.
5. Once the time is almost off, heat your oven up to 450°F.
6. Prepare a baking sheet with foil and brush it with a little bit of olive oil.
7. Remove carefully the bag from the water bath.
8. Remove the readily prepared sunchokes from the bag and let them dry.
9. Smash each of the sunchokes with the heel of the hand, so they must be about 1/2 inch thick.
10. Put the sunchokes on the baking sheet, sprinkle with remaining olive oil. Season with pepper and salt.
11. Roast the sunchokes a little bit until the edges are a little bit crisp and get the golden color. It takes usually 20 minutes.
12. Spread the almonds over the sunchokes and continue roasting for some minutes more.
13. Remove the sunchokes to a serving plate.
14. Garnish with chives.
15. Bon Appetite!

Sous Vide Vegan Cauliflower Alfredo

The silky and thick texture of the cauliflower will charm you from the first taste! This dish could be eaten for breakfast or as an additional dish to meat in the late evening.

Ingredients (8 servings):

4 cups	cauliflower
2 cups	water
2/3 cup	cashews
2 cloves	garlic
1/2 teaspoon	oregano, dried
1/2 teaspoon	basil, dried
1/2 teaspoon	rosemary, dried
4 tablespoons	nutritional yeast

Salt to taste

pepper at will

Directions:
1. Set the sous vide cooker to 185F.
2. Wash and dry with a paper towel the cauliflower. Cut in florets if it is too large.
3. Peel the garlic and mince it.
4. Add water, cauliflower, cashews, minced garlic, dried oregano, rosemary and basil to a seal bag and close.
5. Put the bag into the sous vide and let it cook for 1 1/2 – 2 hours.
6. Pour contents into your blender. Add salt and pepper at will.
7. Serve warm. Dress with your favorite sauce.
8. Bon Appetite!

Sous vide vegan curry-carrot soup

This yellow curry-carrot vegan soup is an amazing dish on hot summer days. Using the sous vide method all the ingredients will save their vitamins and minerals.

Ingredients (servings):

1 pound	carrots
1 cup	unsweetened coconut milk
1 stalk	lemongrass
1 pcs	shallot, thinly sliced
1 tablespoon	Thai red chili paste
2 teaspoons	kosher salt
2 teaspoons	yellow curry powder
1 teaspoon	ground turmeric
1 clove	garlic

Pepper and salt if desired

Directions:

1. Wash the carrots. Peel and sliced carefully into ½-inch slices.
2. Set the sous vide cooker to 190F.
3. Slice lemongrass into 2-inch pieces also.
4. Peel the garlic and mince. Peel and slice the shallot.
5. Put into seal bag minced garlic, add ground turmeric, kosher salt, curry powder, carrots, lemongrass, shallots. Add also chili paste.
6. Close the bag and set the time for 1 -1,5 hours.
7. Once the time is off, remove the sealed bag.
8. Remove the lemongrass and pour the rest to the blender. Puree the ingredients ca. 1-2 minutes until smooth.
9. Add the coconut milk to reach the necessary consistency.
10. Season with salt and pepper at will.
11. Bon Appetite!

Sous Vide Turmeric Tofu with Lime

One of my favorite vegetarian recipes is Tofu with lime. It is a wonderful combination of soy cheese and green lime that must be also cooked by you!

Ingredients (7 servings):

1 (15-ounce) package	firm Tofu
2 tablespoon	olive oil
4 cloves	garlic
2 teaspoons	ground black pepper
1 teaspoon	ground turmeric
1 teaspoon	kosher salt
2 pcs	limes

Salt and pepper at will

Directions:
1. Open the bag with a firm piece of Tofu and slice into big blocks.
2. Take a medium-sized skillet and roast a little bit the Tofu slices for some minutes until they become a golden color.
3. Peel the garlic and mince.
4. Wash limes and cut into wedges.
5. Set the sous vide cooker to 190F.
6. Take a small bowl, conjoin olive oil, garlic, turmeric, and salt. Add pepper at will.
7. Put the Tofu in a single layer in a sealed bag. Drizzle the tofu with the garlic-turmeric mixture finely.
8. Seal the bag and set the timer for 2 hours.
9. Once the preparation time is almost off, heat a medium-sized skillet.
10. Remove the bag from the water bath.
11. Remove the tofu from the bag, put in on the baking sheet, covered with parchment paper.
12. Drizzle the rest oil over the tofu.
13. Roast until browned, approximately 2 minutes per side.
14. Transfer to a serving plate.
15. Squeeze the lime juice over tofu.
16. Eat warm!

Sous vide Brussels sprouts

This recipe of the Brussels sprouts is especially flavor and delicious in a combination with cashews. You may also add the other nuts as you wish.

Ingredients (7 servings):

16 pcs   Brussels sprouts

1.5-pound   sprout top

2 pcs   bay leaves

1 cup   miso paste

½ cup   unsalted butter

½ cup   cashew nuts

1 tbsp   tarragon leaves

Directions:
1. Set the sous vide cooker to 190F.
2. Put miso paste into a small and add the butter. Conjoin everything well.
3. Remove the hard stalks from the sprout tops.
4. Chop the roasted cashews.
5. Put the sprouts into a sealed bag, add bay leaves and half of the miso butter ready-made.
6. Close the seal and put into the bath for 50 minutes.
7. Put the sprout tops into another sealed bag along. Add there also the remained butter. Close and put into the water bath. Cook for 20-25 minutes.
8. Remove the sprouts on a plate and add cashews and tarragon leaves.
9. Bon Appetite!

Squash and rosemary terrine, chestnut and vacherin

Flavor, simply, delicious side or main dish is for those who are vegetarian. It has an amazing texture and tastes great!

Ingredients (5 servings):

1 pcs	butternut squash
½ cup	unsalted butter
2 tbsp	rosemary
salt	
½ cup	vacherin
4 pcs	fresh chestnuts

fresh tarragon if desired

Directions:

1. Set the sous vide cooker to 190F.
2. Wash and peel the squash. Slice it vertically into 2mm pieces, after this slice into rectangles.
3. Wash and chop the rosemary.
4. Put the butter into a skillet, dress finely with salt and the rosemary.
5. Keep stirring over high heat. Wait until butter will melt.
6. Cover each of squash slice with the butter mixture, just lay the mix on the top of it.
7. After each piece of squash is fully covered with butter, put them to the sealed bag.
8. Pour the rest of butter into the bag and close with the vacuum sealer.
9. Prepare the squash sous vide for 50 minutes
10. Let the squash cool or refrigerate for some hours.
11. After this procedure, take off the squash and heat oil in a little skillet.
12. Slice the squash into some number of servings and put it to the skillet.
13. Roast a little bit from each side, add the rosemary butter to the skillet and spoon it on the top of each serving.
14. Transfer the servings to a plate and add some vacherin cheese on top.
15. Sprinkle some chestnuts on top.
16. Drizzle the butter over the squash pieces and add the tarragon.
17. Bon Appetite!

Sous vide beetroot in beef dripping and pomegranate molasses

Smoked beetroot tastes great in a combination with flavor pomegranate molasses, lemon zest, and thyme. The technique sous vide makes the beetroot more satiated as usual.

Ingredients (5 servings):

500 lb   young beetroots

1 cup   beef dripping

2 tbsp   pomegranate molasses

2 sprigs   thyme

½ cup   lemon zest

Pomegranate seeds

Salt and black pepper at will

Directions:

1. Set the sous vide cooker to 190F.
2. Wash the beetroot, peel, and cut in halves.
3. Prepare the beetroot inside the BBQ. Let it smoke for 35 minutes and then set aside. Let it cool.
4. Put the beetroot into a bowl, add slowly molasses, thyme, zest. Melt the beef dripping and add it also.
5. Add the lemon zest, dress with salt and pepper. Toss everything together.
6. Let the beetroot be prepared sous vide for 3-3,5 hours until the wished firmness.
7. Once the time is over, remove the beetroot and let it dry.
8. Put a pan on to a high or medium-high heat, and let the beetroot caramelize a little.
9. Serve hot and dress with black pepper and thyme.
10. Bon Appetite!

Pork and Beef

Sous vide pork chops

This is a classic recipe of pork chops prepared in the sous vide. This time you need to have only three (!) main components such as meat, butter and oil and you'll get an amazing essential meal for a whole day!

Ingredients (3 ingredients):

2 pcs	Pork Chops
1 tbsp	Vegetable Oil
1 tbsp	Butter

Rosemary or thyme if desired

Pepper and salt at will

Directions:

1. Set the sous vide cooker to 140F.
2. Season pork carefully with pepper, add salt. Do this from all the sides.
3. Put pork into the sealed bag. Add rosemary if you wish or thyme if desired.
4. Seal the bag using a vacuum sealer.
5. Drop the bag in the water bath. Let it cook for 2 hours.
6. Once the time is over, take off the pork from the sealed bag. Put it on a plate and let it dry a little. Take off the species.
7. Add vegetable oil, butter to the large skillet and set it in a high heat. Wait until the butter is melted.
8. Put the pork chops into the skillet. Let it cook until the crust is a deep brown. It takes 1 minute usually. Do the same from both sides.
9. Once the pork gets a golden color, take off the skillet and remove the pork chops on a plate.
10. Slice the pork chops before serving. Season with pepper and salt added.
11. Bon Appetite!

Sous vide pork tenderloin

There is the best recipe of the pork tenderloin I've ever tried! Use your favorite fresh herbs, shallots, and garlic.

Ingredients (6 servings):

1 pound	Pork Tenderloin
6 to 8 Sprigs	Fresh Herbs at will
2 cloves	Garlic
2 pcs	shallots
1 tbsp	vegetable oil
1 tbsp	butter

Pepper and salt if desired

Directions:

1. Set the sous vide cooker to 140F.
2. Season pork carefully with pepper, add salt. Do this from all the sides.
3. Peel the shallots. Slice them.
4. Peel the garlic and mince it.
5. Put pork into the seal bag. Add fresh herbs.
6. Seal the bag using a vacuum sealer. Drop the bag in the water bath. Let it cook for 4 hours.
7. Once the time is over, take off the pork from the seal bag. Put it on a plate and let it dry a little. Save the juice from the sealed bag in a separate cup or deep plate.
8. Heat the oil in a large skillet, add pork and cook it for 1-2 minutes from all the sides if you want to get the golden color of pork. Remove the pork from a plate and set them aside.
9. Add to the same skillet shallots, garlic, species, and butter. Add the remained juice from the sealed bag if desired.
10. Once shallots are caramelized, remove the skillet from a heat and pour the mix over the pork slices in a plate.
11. Serve hot. Add salt and pepper if desired.
12. Bon Appetite!

Sous vide pork loin with cumin crust, grilled asparagus, and lemon

Sous vide pork covered fully with Dijon mustard and cumin tastes great with tomatoes, cucumbers, eggplants. This is a great recipe for parties and family dinners!

Ingredients (10 servings):

1 ½ lb	pork loin
4 tbsp	Dijon Mustard
4 tbsp	Cumin Seeds
1 tbsp	Dried Oregano
1 tbsp	Smoked Paprika
1 tsp	Mustard Powder
2 pcs	Lemon
½ cup	Breadcrumbs
½ cup	Parmesan
2 Bunch	Asparagus

Olive Oil

Salt and pepper to taste

Directions:
1. Peel the asparagus and wash.
2. Take a small bowl, add paprika and cumin. Add also lemon zest, add mustard powder and a little bit oregano. Add the sea salt. Add pepper.
3. Season the pork with a little bit mustard.
4. Grate Parmesan and set aside.
5. Put the pork in a sealed bag, seal and let it cook sous vide for 4-5 hours under 130F.
6. In another bowl, mix the crumbs with the grated Parmesan. Season with salt
7. Take a little skillet, add oil and add asparagus and saute until golden color.
8. Once the cooking time is over, remove the pork from the sealed bag, cover with mustard. Cover the pork slices in the crumb mix from all the sides carefully.
9. Roast the meat in a large skillet for some minutes from both sides.
10. Serve on a plate adding grilled asparagus and cumin seeds.
11. Bon Appetite!

Sous vide Barbeque pork recipe

You prepare the Barbeque pork using the sous vide technique at any time and you don't need to go outside and search for a fire. Tender meat an in flavor sauce is an amazing variation for summer holidays and weekends.

Ingredients (15 servings):

1 cup	ketchup
1/4 cup	apple cider vinegar
2 tablespoons	yellow mustard
2 tablespoons	brown sugar
1 tablespoon	Worcestershire sauce
1/2 teaspoon	onion powder
1/2 teaspoon	garlic powder
1/2 teaspoon	dried oregano
1/2 teaspoon	paprika
1/2 teaspoon	chili powder
1/8 teaspoon	cayenne pepper
2 1/2 teaspoons	salt
1 1/2 teaspoons	pepper at will
4 pounds	boneless pork shoulder
2 tablespoons	canola oil

Directions:
1. Set the sous vide cooker to 140F.
2. Cut the pork shoulders into pieces. Season carefully with pepper, add salt. Do this from all the sides. Set aside.
3. Take a bowl of medium-size, add ketchup and vinegar, mustard, brown sugar. Toss everything well.
4. Add Worcestershire sauce, onion and garlic powder, oregano, paprika, chili powder, cayenne pepper. Stir everything.
5. Put the meat slices in a sealed bag and pour the sauce. Once you close the bag, make a light massage to a bag of meat. Let the sous spread over the meat.
6. Put the bags in a water bath and let it cook for 4 hours.

7. Once the time is over, remove the bags, open them and take off the meat on a plate. Put the pieces on a baking sheet, sprinkle with oil. Grill at 400F up to 5 minutes in general from all the sides.
8. Serve immediately!
9. Bon Appetite!

Sous vide Teriyaki Pork

This pork prepared in a Teriyaki sauce could be served with rice or noodles or some vegetable salad.

Ingredients (5 servings):

1 pound	whole pork tenderloin
2 tbsp	salted butter
1 tbsp	olive oil
1 cup	Teriyaki sauce
½ cup	mustard sauce

Pepper and salt at will

Directions:
1. Set the sous vide cooker to 140F.
2. Cut salted butter in three slices.
3. Cover pork with Teriyaki sauce.
4. In a sealed bag put the whole pork in a sauce and place three pieces of butter.
5. Close the sealed bag and cook 2-3 hours.
6. Once the time is over, open the bag, remove the pork and set aside. Save the liquid from the bag in a small bowl.
7. Take a little skillet, add olive oil. Slice the pork.
8. In a small bowl with the rest of the liquid the Teriyaki sauce again, add mustard sauce. Pour over the meat slices and roast them for some minutes in a skillet from both sides.
9. Serve hot!
10. Bon Appetite!

Sous vide medium-rare steak

This recipe of sous vide beef is only for those who like medium rare consistency. The meat will be of light red color inside.

Ingredients (2 servings):

1 (8- to 12-ounce)   boneless tenderloin

1 tbsp   olive oil

salt and black pepper

Directions:
1. Set the sous vide cooker to 140F.
2. Prepare the steak – season it gently with salt. Add pepper. Put it in a sealed bag. Close it. Put the bag in the water bath. Let it cook for 2 hours.
3. Once the time is off, remove the bag from the water bath.
4. Take off the steak from the bag. Let it dry a little bit.
5. Take a medium-sized skillet, heat the olive oil.
6. Put meat into a heated skillet, roast it for some minutes from all the sides.
7. Transfer the steak into a plate and cut it.
8. Serve hot.

Sous vide beef and prune tagine

The best way of cooking this recipe of beef with prunes is sous vide. Finally, you'll get tender meat with an unusual combination of tastes. Don't hesitate to cook it!

Ingredients (12 servings):

1 pound	beef
2 pcs	onions
1 pinch	saffron
1 tsp	ground ginger
1 tsp	ground cinnamon
1 tsp	garlic powder
½ cup	prunes
1 tbsp	honey
50g of	butter
5 pcs	ice cubes
1 tbsp	olive oil
Salt, pepper	
½ cup	couscous for serving

Directions:

1. Preheat the water bath to 135F.
2. Cut the beef into medium-sized cubes.
3. Peel and chop onions finely.
4. Season the beef with pepper.
5. Take a large pan, heat the oil and roast the beef there. The sides of the beef must get light golden color. Set aside.
6. To the same pan add onions, wait until they will be caramelized. Add oil if necessary.
7. Put the meat into seal bag, add saffron and onions. Add ginger and cinnamon. Add also garlic, prunes. Distribute all the ingredients in a sealed bag.
8. Add honey. Add also butter, put the ice cubes.
9. Close and leave for approximately 11 hours.
10. Once the time is over, remove meat from the bag, slice at will.
11. Serve with couscous. Pour the liquid over the top of meat. Garnish with coriander.
12. Bon Appetite!

Sous Vide Red Curry Crusted Beef

Simply clever recipe of beef steaks with cucumber mix. This is a must-try dish with a special Asian flavor.

Ingredients (11 servings):
For the Steaks

2 Pieces	Beef Rib Steaks
2 Tbsp	Curry Paste
Salt if desired	

For the mix

1.5 Cups	Cucumber
1 Cup	radish
1 Piece	Red Thai Chili
1 bunch	Basil
1 bunch	Mint
2 Cloves	garlic
1 Tbsp	Honey
1 Tbsp	Fish Sauce
1 Tbsp	Tamarind Paste

Directions:
1. Wash and slice the cucumbers.
2. Wash and slice radish.
3. Finely and carefully chop chili.
4. Wash and chop finely basil and mint.
5. Peel and mince garlic.
6. In a small bowl mix together honey, chili, fish sauce, tamarind. Toss everything well. Add mint, basil.
7. Combine everything with radish and cucumber.
8. Spread the curry paste over the meat. Put it into a seal bag and close.
9. Let it cook for 50 minutes at 125F.
10. Once the cooking time is over, transfer the beef to a skillet, add a little bit oil and roast meat from all the sides if desired.
11. Serve immediately with cucumbers mix.
12. Bon Appetite!

Sous vide Greek burgers with Feta

Vary your usual burgers with this new taste of the Mediterranean. Everybody likes burgers, so do I. Try to cook the burgers on my recipe!

Ingredients (13 servings):
For the Patties

1 pound	Ground Beef
1 Tbsp	Marjoram
1 Tbsp	Oregano
1 Tbsp	Parsley Flakes
1 Tbsp	Salt
1/2 Tbsp	Black Pepper

For the Feta Cream

2/3 Cup	Heavy Cream
1/2 Cup	Feta
1/2 Tbsp	Garlic Powder
1 Tsp	Pepper
1/2 Tsp	Salt

For Serving

2 Pieces	Burger Buns
1 Piece	Red Onion

Lettuce

Directions:
Preparing the patties:

1. In a deep bowl mix ground beef, marjoram, parsley, oregano, salt. Form the patties using your hands.
2. Put the patties into seal bags. Let it cook at 140F ca. 45 minutes.
3. Prepare the Feta cream: in a large bowl mix egg yolks and cream. Whisk together. Slice Feta. Add to the mixture. Also add garlic powder, salt, and pepper.
4. Once the patties are ready, put them to an ice bath.
5. Sear patties in a hot skillet for a minute from each side.

6. Slice the burgers in a middle, sliced red onion. Add Feta cream, lettuce, onion slices, and fresh parsley and patties.
7. Bon Appetite!

Sous Vide Steak Japanese Style

Cooking steak in Japanese style using the method of sous vide you don't need to attend high-quality Japanese restaurants and lose your money! Today it is possible to prepare this dish at home! You can find here the necessary ingredients and simple directions on how to cook it.

Ingredients (7 servings):

1 clove	garlic
1 1-thick (2.5 cm)	steak
1 Tbsp	olive oil for sous vide preparation
1 Tbsp	vegetable oil
1 pcs	green onion
1-inch	daikon
1-2 Tbsp	ponzu

Pepper and salt at will

Directions:
1. Preheat the water bath to 135F.
2. Peel and mince the garlic.
3. Peel and slice the onion.
4. Sprinkle meat with salt. Add black pepper if desired.
5. Put the steak in the bag. Put garlic slices. Add olive oil.
6. Vacuum the sealed bag and let it cook for 4 hours.
7. Grate the daikon.
8. Once the time is over, remove the steak from the bag, let it dry a little. Take off the slices of garlic.
9. Take a large skillet, add oil, place on high heat. Sear each side of steaks ca. 1-2 minutes until golden crust. After it is done, cut the steak into small ½ inch pieces.
10. Squeeze the grated daikon and put it on a top of the steak pieces.
11. Spread the green onion and pour the ponzu on each small slice.
12. Enjoy warm.
13. Bon Appetite!

Poultry

Sous vide chicken breast

I like this recipe of chicken sous vide because the variations how to combine the ready-made chicken are great! You may serve it with different sauces, vegetables, mayo, and herbs.

Ingredients (2 servings):

1 pound   chicken breast

1 tbsp   Vegetable oil

Salt and pepper at will

Fresh herbs (optional)

Lemon slices (optional)

Directions
1. Preheat the water bath to 135F.
2. Wash the chicken breasts, season with salt. Add pepper if desired.
3. Wash the lemon and slice finely.
4. Put the chicken breasts into a sealed bag, add herbs and lemon slices.
5. Close the sealed bag. Put in the water bath and cook for 1-1.5 hours.
6. Once the time is over, take off the chicken, remove the lemon slices and the rest of herbs.
7. Put the skillet on a medium heat, add oil.
8. Carefully put the chicken into the skillet and press with hand.
9. Roast carefully from both sides. Take it off from the skillet once it is done.
10. Take off the wishbone and slice.
11. Season with favorite herbs, lemon slices or desired vegetables.
12. Bon Appetite!

Sous vide chicken wings

To cook this simple recipe you need only three ingredients – chicken wings, salt, and oil. The rest work will do your sous vide! Serve the chicken wings hot with chili or ketchup!

Ingredients (3 servings):

10 pcs   chicken wings

1 pinch   salt

½ cup   vegetable oil

Pepper at will

Directions:

1. Preheat the water bath to a temperature of 135F.
2. Wash the chicken wings. Dive all the wings into three sections. Slice them through the joints.
3. Season the slices with salt. Add pepper at will.
4. Put the wings inside the seal bag and close.
5. Leave it at the water bath for 5 hours.
6. Take off the wing once the time is over.
7. Roast them in a medium-sized skillet, adding oil until crisp
8. Serve immediately!
9. Bon Appetite!

Spiced chicken thighs, charred spring onions, and lime

Amazing, quick, flavor, simple recipe of chicken thighs. You may cook it both for family supper or night party!

Ingredients (7 servings):

4 large thighs	chicken thighs
1 tbsp.	harissa spice
½ zest	lemon
2 sprigs	thyme
1 tsp	garlic powder
1 bunch	spring onions
1 pcs	lime

Salt and pepper at will

Directions:
1. Preheat the water bath to a temperature of 135F.
2. Wash the chicken thighs. Put them onto a plate. Season with harissa, lemon zest. Add thyme and garlic powder. Don't forget about salt and pepper (at will).
3. Put the chicken thighs inside the seal bag and close.
4. Leave it at the water bath for 5 hours.
5. Take off the thighs once the time is over. Let them dry a little.
6. Out the saucepan on a high heat. Add oil, put the chicken thighs. Fry them until golden color.
7. Wash and cut spring onions. Add to the saucepan with thighs. Add some lime juice.
8. Serve hot!
9. Bon Appetite!

Sous vide whole chicken

Flavor chicken that is cooked with thyme, olive oil, and stock cube. Tender structure of meat could be mixed with ripe tomatoes, bell peppers and other vegetables you prefer.

Ingredients (4 servings):

1 – 1 ½   Chicken

1 cube   Chicken Stock

1 tsp   Thyme

1 tbsp   Olive Oil

Salt and pepper at will

Directions:
1. Wash the chicken thoroughly. Cut out the backbone.
2. Press down on the breasts to flatten.
3. Preheat the water bath to a temperature of 135F.
4. Brush chicken carefully with olive oil.
5. Crumble finely the stock cube over the chicken.
6. Add thyme.
7. Put the chicken inside the seal bag and close.
8. Leave it at the water bath for 4 hours.
9. Take off the chicken once the time is over. Let them dry a little.
10. Bake in the oven for 7 minutes until skin is crisp.
11. Serve on a big plate!

Sous vide goose breast with blackberries

There many different variations of meat with berries – sauce from berries or just like berries as an addition to the main dish. This time I would like to present you my variation of meat cooked sous vide in a delicious unusual combination with sweet blackberries.

Ingredients (12 servings)

2 x 400g	Goose Breasts
1 tbsp	Brown Sugar
2 tbsp	Treacle
2 tsp	Thyme
10 pcs	Juniper Berries
1 pcs	Bay Leaf
3 Cloves	garlic
2 Bags	Hibiscus Tea
150mls	Sloe Gin
1 tbsp	Castor Sugar
1 pcs	Orange (zest)
1 cup	Blackberries

Salt and pepper at will

Directions:
1. Take a medium-sized bowl and conjoin treacle, juniper, tea, add bay leaf, salt, sloe gin. Mix everything thoroughly.
2. Peel the garlic and mince it. Add also to a bowl.
3. Take a medium-sized skillet, pour the mixture from bowl to the skillet and saute a little bit.
4. Wash the goose breasts, take off the skin. Take a saucepan and render the fat of the breast.
5. Pour the ready-made brine through the sieve.
6. Put the breast into the bowl with brine and place into the fridge for a night.
7. Cover berries with castor sugar, sole Gin, add the orange zest. Set aside.
8. Put goose breast in a sealed bag, close and cook for 3 hours under 140F.
9. Remove the breast from the bag, fry it a little in a skillet. Try to caramelize it from both sides.
10. Serve hot with marinated blackberries.
11. Bon Appetite!

Sous vide turkey breasts

Cooking turkey breasts sous vide you'll get perfectly tasty meat that you may serve for family supper, dinner or parties with fresh veggies and sauces.

Ingredients (2 servings):

1 pcs   trimmed turkey breast

1 tbsp   olive oil

Salt and pepper at will

Favorite herbs if desired

Directions:
1. Set the temperature of the water bath for 140F.
2. Wash the meat. Season it with species if desired. Add salt and pepper.
3. Put it to the sealed bag, close and let it cook for 3 hours.
4. Once the time is over, take off the meat, let it dry a little.
5. Preheat a medium-sized pan. Add olive oil and fry the meat skin side. The skin must be crisp. Remove to a plate.
6. Serve hot.
7. Bon appetite!

Sous vide boned and rolled turkey leg

The rolled turkey leg with delicious and flavor species, aroma honey, nutmeg, dried apricots and clementine zest is an amazing creation to surprise your guests.

Ingredients (11 servings):

2 pcs	Turkey Legs, bone removed
4 pcs	zest of a clementine
¼ tsp	Nutmeg
¼ tsp	Mixed Spice (choose your favorite spice)
½ cup	Dried Apricots
3 tbsp	Honey
10 pcs	Sage Leaves
2 Cubes	Chicken Stock
8 pcs	Juniper Berries
5 tbsp	Cranberry Sauce
½ cup	Butter

Pepper and salt at will

Directions:
1. Prepare flavored butter – mix the chosen species with honey, chopped sage.
2. Chop finely the dried apricots. Add nutmeg to the mix.
3. Blend the mix thoroughly.
4. Lay the turkey leg skin side down on a large sheet, season with pepper and salt, some species.
5. Add the clementine zest. Pour the cranberry sauce.
6. Put the butter into the center of the turkey. Roll it carefully.
7. Put the turkey into seal bag, add chicken stock and cook for 7 hours under 135F.
8. Once the cooking time is over, take off the turkey leg. Let it dry a little.
9. Serve with crushed juniper berries.
10. Bon Appetite!

Sous vide tequila chicken

The tequila chicken prepared in technique sous vide is a delicious and flavor that must be eaten hot. A glass of red wine will be a great addition to this dish!

Ingredients (4 servings):

2 pcs   chicken breast halves, boneless and skinless

2 tablespoons   butter

2 tablespoons   tequila

1 pcs   lime, for juice

Fresh chives at will

Directions:
1. Preheat your water bath to 63.5C.
2. Wash the chicken breasts, dress with salt. Add pepper at will.
3. Put the chicken breasts into a sealed bag, close and let it cook for 2-3 hours.
4. Once the time is over, take off the chicken breasts. Take a medium-sized frypan, add butter and fry quickly the breasts from all the sides.
5. Add to the frypan tequila and deglaze the frypan.
6. Remove the chicken breasts on a plate, squeeze the lime and pour the tequila sauce from the frypan.
7. Serve hot!
8. Bon Appetite!

Sous vide coq au vin

The recipe for this chicken prepared with red wine, vegetables, and species is great. The meat is extremely tender, full of flavor and juice!

Ingredients (11 servings)

1 pcs	chicken
1 bottle	red wine
4 cloves	garlic
10 pcs	shallots
200g	smoked lardons
1 cup	chicken stock
	sprigs of thyme
4 pcs	bay leaves
	Fresh parsley at will
	Sea salt and black pepper if desired
3 tbsp	Olive oil
3 pcs	large carrots
3 stalks	celery stalks
2 tbsp	flour

Directions:
1. Wash the chicken and wash with a paper towel.
2. Peel the garlic and press it.
3. Peel and dice carrots. Finely chop the celery stalks.
4. Mix in a saucepan wine, garlic, smoked lardons. Add stock, bay, carrots, and celery. Let everything simmer a little bit. Set aside and let it cool.
5. Peel the onions. Take another little skillet, melt the butter and soften the onions.
6. Preheat your sous vide to 140F. Put the chicken into the sealed bag, add thyme and cooked onions. Pour the sauce also. Distribute it carefully. Let it cook for 10 hours.
7. Once the time is over, take off the chicken, save the liquid. Take off the thyme.
8. Take a saucepan, add red wine, butter, flour and mix well all the time until combined. Add pepper and salt if needed. Let it simmer a little.
9. Place the chicken into the oven and let until crispy. Take off the chicken after some time, pour the mix over the chicken and return back for 2 minutes.

10. Once done, slice the hot meat and serve!
11. Bon Appetite!

Chicken with 40 cloves of garlic

This recipe is better to serve with rice, potatoes or some other vegetables. The hardest work here – is to peel the garlic cloves! Enjoy this dish with me today!

Ingredients (5 servings):

8 pcs   chicken leg quarters

3 tbsp   olive oil

4 sprigs   thyme

2 sprigs   rosemary

40 cloves   garlic

Pepper and salt at will

Directions:
1. Preheat your water bath to 176F.
2. Peel the garlic cloves.
3. Wash the chicken.
4. Season chicken with salt. Put into seal bag.
5. Add olive oil (a half of it), rosemary, garlic, thyme. Close the seal bag. Let it cook for 6 hours or more.
6. After preparation time is over, preheat the frypan, add the rest oil, remove the legs from the sealed bag and put into frypan. Cook 3-4 minutes from each side until crisp.
7. Serve hot.
8. Bon Appetite!

Sous vide chicken with English mustard

Sous vide chicken thighs prepared on this recipe could be eaten with side dishes or as a simple dish for dinner, supper or even breakfast!

Ingredients (10 servings):

6 pcs	chicken thighs
6 slices	lemon
1 pcs	golden onion
1 tbsp	English mustard
2 tbsp	butter
2 tbsp	plain flour
½ cup	white wine
1 cup	light chicken or vegetable stock
3 tbsp	cream cheese
3 tbsp	Olive oil

Sea salt

Black pepper at will

Directions:

1. Preheat the bath to 170F.
2. Wash the chicken thighs and season with pepper. Add salt.
3. Slice the lemon and squeeze the juice, spread over the thighs, add olive oil on the pieces and toss with hands in a large bowl.
4. Put the thighs into the seal bag, close. Put into the water bath for 1,5 hour.
5. Once the preparation time is over, take off the thighs, let them cool a little.
6. Meanwhile use another large bowl mix flour, melted butter, wine, mustard, stock. Whisk until smooth consistency. Let the mix simmer in a medium-sized skillet.
7. Put the thighs (without juice) into the skillet, toss carefully in the mix. Add cream cheese and sliced onions.
8. Fry for 3-4 minutes. Toss thighs all the time.
9. Serve hot with fresh bread.
10. Bon Appetite!

Eggs

Sous Vide Egg Bites: Bacon & Gruyere

These egg bites are so easy to prepare – add bacon slices and grated gruyere and you'll get amazing breakfast!

Ingredients (5 servings):

6 pcs	eggs
1/2 cup	gruyere
1/4 cup	cream cheese
1/4 tsp	salt
3 slices	bacon

Directions:
1. Set sous vide for 172ºF.
2. Cut the bacon in halves.
3. Grate cheese.
4. Take a blender, conjoin eggs, cheese, salt. Add finely pepper at will and whisk until smooth.
5. Take the jars, put them on a surface. Place bacon slices inside, pour the mix in each jar. Close.
6. Put them in a heated bath and let them cook for 1 hour.
7. Once the time is over, take off the jars, so you may eat straight from it or push it carefully to a plate!
8. Bon Appetite!

Sous Vide Soft-Poached Eggs

Ingredients (1 servings):

1-16 large eggs

Salt and pepper

Directions

1. Set the sous vide for 172ºF.
2. Put eggs into a heat bath. Cover and let it cook for 10 minutes.
3. Take a large bowl and fill it with ice. Use the long spoon to take the eggs and put them in the bowl with ice. Cool 1 minute.
4. Crack eggs right before eating. Add salt.
5. Bon Appetite!

Sous Vide Bacon and Jarlsberg Egg Bite

There is a light mix of eggs, bacon, cream cheeses and hard cheese. Add your favorite species and your simple delicious breakfast is ready!

Ingredients (8 servings):

6 pcs	Eggs
1/2 cup	Cheese Jarlsberg
4 oz	Bacon
1/2 cup	Cream Cheese
1/4 cup	Heavy Cream
1 teaspoon	Salt
1 pinch	Black Pepper
1 Tbsp	Butter

Directions:
1. Take a little frypan and roast bacon.
2. Take a bowl, whisk eggs, heavy cream, cheese, pepper, salt. Whisk until smooth consistency. Divide into jars.
3. Spread grated cheese. Add bacon.
4. Put in the heat bath and let them cook for 1 hour.
5. Once the time is over, take off the jars from the bath, so you may eat straight from it or push it carefully to a plate!
6. Bon Appetite!

Sous Vide Eggs Benedict Pizza Recipe

The benedict pizza is a classic breakfast. This time I have used traditional components in an unusual combination of techniques. This dish is perfect for any morning brunch.

Ingredients (8 servings):

1 pcs   Pizza Dough

3 pcs   Eggs

2 oz.   mozzarella

3 slices   Canadian bacon

 1 tbsp   Hollandaise Sauce

fresh Parsley

Hollandaise Sauce

2 pcs   egg yolks

½ pcs   lemon

salt

cayenne pepper

1/2 stick   butter

Directions:

1. Take a bowl and conjoin egg yolks, juice from the lemon, salt and whisk together. Add pepper.
2. Melt the butter. Add to the sauce and whisk all together once more.
3. Preparing the eggs - Set sous vide to 170 F, put eggs carefully. Cook for 10 minutes, then take them off. Place in cold water. Set aside.
4. Cook the pizza – preheat the oven to 500F.
5. Roll the dough to around, dust finely with flour.
6. Put fresh mozzarella, slices of bacon on the top. Place it on a baking sheet and cook for 3-4 minutes in the oven.
7. Take off the pizza, crack the eggs that you have cooked sous vide (they must be on a top). Add pepper and salt at will.
8. Sprinkle with sauce over the eggs.
9. Enjoy warm! Use fresh parsley for serving.
10. Bon Appetite!

Sauce, stock, and broth

Cranberry sauce cooked sous vide

To prepare this flavor colorful sauce you may you both fresh and frozen cranberries. If you use frozen cranberries, let them dry before cooking and remove unnecessary liquid from the bag.

Ingredients (3 servings):

½ cup   cranberries

3 tbsp   sugar

½ pcs   orange zest

Directions:
1. Wash the cranberries. Let them dry finely.
2. Put two water baths rests. Place the dried cranberries between two steps.
3. Put sugar, berries, and zest into seal bag and close. Put it into heat bath under 170F for 2 hours.
4. Once the time is over, let the cranberries cool.
5. Pour the sauce into a bowl before serving.
6. Bon Appetite!

Hollandaise sauce sous vide

While cooking the hollandaise it could split when using the high temperature. But if you cook these amazing sauce sous vide – no problems will arise!

Ingredients (6 servings):

¼ cup   white wine vinegar

1 pcs   shallots

5 tbsp   butter

5 pcs   egg yolks

¼ cup   water

2 tbsp   lemon juice

Salt at will

Directions:
1. Set the water bath to 170F.
2. Peel the shallots and slice. In a little frypan roast the shallots in butter for some minutes. Add wine vinegar.
3. Put egg yolk, salt, lemon juice, butter, cooked shallots in the sealed bag and close.
4. Put it into heat bath for 1 hour.
5. Once the time is over, you may use the sauce at once taking it off from the sealed bag. If not leave it in a water bath by temperature 150F for some time.
6. Bon Appetite!

Hot sauce sous vide

This spicy homemade sauce is a great addition to beef, poultry, goose or pork. You may use also another pepper, for example, hot chili.

Ingredients (4 servings):

0,5-pound   jalapeño peppers

9 clove   garlic

sea salt

3 tbsp   rice vinegar

2 tbsp   simple syrup

Directions:
1. Set the water oven to 170F.
2. Wash the peppers, take off the seeds, chop finely. Be careful as they are hot.
3. Peel the garlic and mince.
4. Put peppers and garlic into a blender. Mix well.
5. Put the pure into the sealed bag. Close and let it cook for 25 minutes.
6. Transfer the mixture to a bowl, add vinegar and syrup.
7. Refrigerate for some hours.
8. Bon Appetite!

Mango chutney sous vide

This is the most flavor sauce and addition to all the meals! It is beautiful and full of fruits and vegetables! Don't hesitate to cook it today!

Ingredients (13 servings):

3 pcs	mango
3 tbsp	olive oil
3 pcs	red chili flakes
1 tbsp	pineapple juice
1 tbsp	cider vinegar
3 tbsp	brown sugar
1 tsp	curry powder
1/4 tsp	salt
1/8 tsp	white pepper
1 pcs	red onion
1 tsp	fresh ginger
1 pcs	red bell pepper
2 tbsp	raisins

Directions:
1. Set the water bath to 182F.
2. Wash and peel the mango. Chop it finely.
3. Peel the onion and dice. Peel and mince ginger.
4. Wash and slice finely bell pepper. Take off the seeds.
5. Chop the raisins.
6. Take a bowl, combine vinegar, pineapple juice, curry, sugar, pepper. Add salt. Mix well.
7. Add oil, pepper flakes and toss together until paste consistency.
8. Put mango, bell pepper, ginger, raisins into the sealed bag, add paste. Add white pepper. Mix everything together. Close and let it cook for 6 hours.
9. Once the time is over, put the seal bag in the ice water for 25 minutes.
10. Refrigerate for some hours.
11. Bon Appetite!

Summer corn salsa sous vide

This hot salsa sous vide is amazing for fish, grilled meat, poultry. You may just eat it with chips.

Ingredients (8 servings):

4 ears   fresh corn

2 cloves   garlic

1 pcs   jalapenos

2 pcs   tomatoes

2 pcs   limes

¼ cup   olive oil

2 pcs   avocados

1 bunch   coriander

Pepper and salt at will

Directions:
1. Set the water bath to 170F.
2. Shuck and wash the corn. Season with salt from all the sides.
3. Put it to the sealed bag, close and let it cook for 1 hour.
4. Peel and mince the garlic.
5. Wash and take off the seeds from jalapenos. Slice.
6. Wash and chop tomatoes.
7. Wash and take off the seed from avocado. Slice finely. Chop coriander.
8. Squeeze juice from lime into a cup.
9. Take a large bowl, conjoin garlic, tomatoes, jalapenos, lime juice, pepper, olive oil, coriander, salt, avocado.
10. Once the corn is ready, remove, let them cool and cut the kernels into a bowl. Toss everything well.
11. Bon Appetite!

Sous vide applesauce

Using the sous vide technique you may cook an amazing applesauce at home! Use only 4 simple ingredients – apples, lemon, cinnamon, and sugar!

Ingredients (4 servings):

4 pcs   apples

1 pcs   lemon

3 tbsp   sugar

½ teaspoon   cinnamon

Directions:

1. Set the water bath to 170F.
2. Wash the apples, peel, take off the seeds, chop finely.
3. Squeeze the juice of lemon, add it to the apple pieces. Mix well in a bowl.
4. Pu the apples to the sealed bag, add cinnamon, sugar. Close and let it cook for 1 hour.
5. Once the time is over, let the mixture cool and pour it into a food processor. Blend to get the smooth sauce.
6. Bon Appetite!

Fresh ginger sauce sous vide

If you want to add a little experiment to your life, prepare the ginger sauce and pour over your favorite ingredients.

Ingredients (4 servings)

½ cup	caster sugar
1 l	water
2-3 pcs	ginger root
½ cup	vodka

Directions:
1. Set the water bath to 170F.
2. Peel the ginger and grate it.
3. Put sugar, ginger into the sealed bag. Add water. Close and let it cook for 1,5 hours.
4. Once the time is over, remove the mix to a bowl, add vodka and toss everything together.
5. Place the pouring sauce into the fridge.
6. You may store it in the fridge up to 2-3 weeks.

Sous vide chicken stock

It is a quite boring and a long thing, to cook the usual stock on the oven. Preparing the chicken stock sous vide allows you to forget about time and difficulties.

Ingredients (8 servings):

2 pounds   chicken bones

2 cups   carrots

2 cups   celery

2 cups   leeks

2 tablespoons   olive oil

8 cups   water

1 tablespoon   black peppercorns

2 pcs   bay leaves

Pepper and salt at will

Directions:
1. Set the water bath to 180°F.
2. Wash carrots, peel and dice. Wash and dice the celery.
3. Wash and dice leeks.
4. Take a bowl, mix chicken bones, celery, carrots, leeks. Add olive oil and toss together. Roast for 15 minutes in a large frypan.
5. Remove the ingredients together with juice to the sealed bag. Add water, peppercorns put the bay leaves. Close and let it cook for 10 hours.
6. Once the time is over, divide the ingredients from the liquid. Pout stock to a large bowl.
7. You may keep it in the fridge for a month.
8. Bon Appetite!

Sous vide beef stock

This flavor stock conjoins beef bones, fresh vegetables, and your favorite species. Let your sous vide technique perform your daily work!

Ingredients (5 servings):

1-pound   beef bones

3 cups   water

1 stick   celery stick

1 pcs   carrot

1 pcs   white onion

Pepper and salt at will

Directions:
1. Set the water bath to 180°F.
2. Wash the celery and chop.
3. Wash carrot and chop finely.
4. Peel the onion and slice.
5. Put beef bones, celery, carrot, onion, salt into the sealed bag. Add pepper and water to it. Close.
6. Let it cook for 12 hours.
7. Once the time is over, divide the ingredients from the liquid. Pout stock to a large bowl.
8. You may keep it in the fridge for a month.
9. Bon Appetite!

Sous vide citrus yogurt

To prepare the own yogurt at home could be so easy! Save money and use the sous vide technique!

Ingredients (5 servings):

1 Liter	Milk
1/2 Cup	Yogurt
1/2 Tbsp	Orange Zest
1/2 Tbsp	Lemon Zest
1/2 Tbsp	Lime Zest

Directions:
1. Heat the milk to 180F in a separate bowl on a stove.
2. Let it cool for 110F.
3. Add yogurt, orange, add lemon and lime zest.
4. Set the water bath to 180°F.
5. Pour it into jars, place into the water bath. Close. Let it cook for 4 hours.
6. Once the time is over, remove from jars from the water.
7. Cool a little and enjoy!
8. Bon Appetite!

Sous vide plumps with red wine

There is an amazing, colorful, cool dessert on a hot sunny day! All the family members and friends will surely like it!

Ingredients (3 servings):

4 Pieces   Plums

1 Cup   Red Wine

1/2 Cup   Sugar

Directions:
1. Set the water bath to 180°F.
2.
3. Wash the plums, cut in halves and remove the seeds.
4. Take a little bowl, pour wine, heat it, add sugar.
5. Put the plumps into the sealed bag, add wine and close the bag.
6. Let it cook for 1 hour.
7. Once the time is over, pour the liquid into a bowl and freeze it.
8. Serve with granita!

Sous Vide Blueberry and Saffron Crème Brûlée

This is a very simple, delicious and fresh creme brulee. Prepare it in a hot summer day. You may refrigerate this dessert and refrigerate for some days or even a week.

Ingredients (5 servings):

2 Cups	Heavy Cream
4 Pieces	Egg Yolks
1/4 Cup	Brown Sugar
1 cup	Blueberries
Pinch	Saffron Threads

Directions:
1. Set the water bath to 180°F.
2. Take a saucepan, heat saffron and cream.
3. Take another saucepan, combine egg yolks and sugar. Whisk everything together.
4. Conjoin egg yolks with heated cream.
5. Prepare the jars, put the blueberries into, pour the mixture into the jars.
6. Close, cook for 1 hour.
7. Once the time is over, let the jars cool for 4 hours.
8. Bon Appetite!

Black Pepper and Mint Sous Vide Pineapples

I'm sure you have never tried an unusual recipe of fresh pineapple cooked sous vide method with salt, fresh flavor mint, and peppercorns!? Eat the ready-made pineapple with ice cream or yogurt.

Ingredients (5 servings):

1 Piece	Pineapple
1/3 Cup	Sugar
1 Tsp	Black Peppercorns
½ cup	Mint

Salt at will

Directions:
1. Set the water bath to 180°F.
2. Wash and peel the pineapple, cut into medium-sized slices.
3. Mix the mint, sugar, salt, peppercorns and toss everything.
4. Coat the slices with mixture. Put the mix into the sealed bag.
5. Let it cook for 1 hour.
6. Once the time is over, remove to a plate!
7. Enjoy cold!

Sous vide vanilla-lemongrass syrup

Let the usual syrups that you prepare almost all the time to get a little bit of flavor. Simple, quick and delicious dessert! Don't hesitate to cook it!

Ingredients (4 servings):

2 Cups	Sugar
1/4 Cup	Water
1 Pod	Vanilla
1 stalk	Lemongrass

Directions:
1. Set the water bath to 190°F.
2. Prepare the lemongrass stalk – bruise with a knife carefully.
3. Take a bowl, conjoin sugar, lemongrass, vanilla and mix everything.
4. Add water. Put the mix into the vacuum bag. Close it and let it cook for 2 hours.
5. Once the time is over, remove the mix and chill in an ice bath.
6. Cool in a refrigerator for some hours and enjoy!

Sous Vide Mango Preserve

This is the simplest preserve I could only imagine! Enjoy colorful, sunny, light mango dessert for your early breakfast!

Ingredients (3 servings):

2 Pieces   Mango

3 Cups   Sugar

1 Piece   Lemon

Directions:

1. Wash and peel the mango. Slice it finely.
2. Take a bowl, mix sugar, mango and lemon juice.
3. Put the mix into the jars, set them to the heated bath.
4. Let it cook for 1 hour at 170F.
5. Once the time is over, remove the jars and let them cool.
6. Bon Appetite!

Conclusion

The cooking method of sous vide has been the utmost secrecy of the great and famous chefs for centuries, giving the food new consistency and accuracy to get the ingredients of high standards. The appliances for the sous vide cooking allow everyone creating gourmet quality meals at home today. The water oven is one of the most unique features with well-engineered design. The exact temperature control allows gaining of both slow and fast changes of the cooking process – slow change of the temperature allows reaching the tender consistency of meat, it could be also pasteurized, so you may keep the ready food in the fridge whole week or even some weeks long. None other methods of cooking allow you extending the shelf-life of products. This process prevents of recontamination of the ingredients during storage. Cooking food using your old methods, the fluid interacts with the ingredients you cook and might wash away all the nutrients. It also affects the texture of products. Sous vide method breaks stereotypes, how long will you cook losing necessary microelements and precious time? It's a high time to change your life and the way you eat. The relative new way of cooking is simply as an alphabet. In the century of high technologies to waste time in a kitchen roasting your steak for an hour is a real crime! Every day we speak about lack of time but still can't manage it... It is a nonsense! Following the easy steps of sous vide method of cooking, everybody can enjoy a healthy and fresh meal full of vitamins and microelements, juicy and colorful; each member of the family can learn the preparations step using the sous vide method, so even your kids will be able to help you in the kitchen. You don't need more unnecessary tools and a lot of accessories in the kitchen. All you need to invest once in the sous vide devices and forget about your problems. I'm sure that cooking sous vide will bring you newest tastes of the well-known ingredients and satisfaction both of the process of cooking and eating!

Author's Afterthoughts

Thanks ever so much to each of my cherished readers for investing the time read this book!

I know you could have picked from many other books but you chose this one. So big thanks for downloading this book and reading all way to the end.

If you enjoyed this book or received value from it, I'd like to ask you for a favor. Please take a few minutes to post an honest and heartfelt review on Amazon.com Your support does make a difference and to benefit other people.

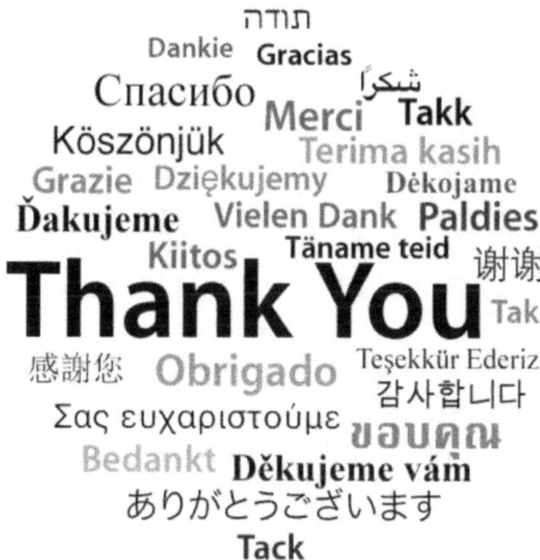

www.ingramcontent.com/pod-product-compliance
Lightning Source LLC
Chambersburg PA
CBHW070040260726
48658CB00002B/678